What do the professionals have to say about logging your important activities?

"Write it down! I guarantee you will want to look back and see how much you have improved."
Tony Horton, creator of *P90X* and author of *Bring It!*

"Eventually runners start keeping a log and then wonder how they ever ran without it."
Jeff Galloway, author of *Galloway's Book of Running*

"Over time, your written log will help you identify strengths, weaknesses, and improvements. You'll be encouraged and inspired when you look back on your log entries and see how far you've come."
Jackie Warner, author of *This is Why You're Fat* and Hollywood personal trainer

"Logs are a great way to track progress and stay motivated."
Margaret Schlachter, author of *Obstacle Race Training*

MUD & OBSTACLE RACE LOGBOOK

+ YOUR RACE LOGBOOK
+ PERFORMANCE TIPS
+ INSPIRATIONAL QUOTES

ROGER D. SMITH

Mud & Obstacle Race Logbook

© Copyright 2015 by Roger Smith. All rights reserved. No part of this book may be reproduced or transmitted in any form or by any means, electronic or mechanical, including photocopying, recording, or by any information storage and retrieval system, without written permission from the author. For information contact Modelbenders.com.

Modelbenders Press books may be purchased for business and promotional use or for special sales. For information please contact the publisher.

PRINTED IN THE UNITED STATES OF AMERICA

Visit our web site at www.modelbenders.com

Designed by Adina Cucicov at Flamingo Designs
Cover image: Tom Legoski

ProBookmark™ is a trademark of Modelbenders LLC.

The Library of Congress has cataloged the paperback edition as follows:

Smith, Roger D.
    Mud & Obstacle Race Logbook/Roger D. Smith. – 2nd ed.
    1. Health & Fitness 2. Exercise 3. Sport
    I. Roger Smith II. Title

ISBN 978-1-938590-05-4

Also by Roger Smith

The New Blueprint for Fitness:
10 Power Habits for Transforming Your Body

Patterns of Strength:
New Habits of Personality, Intelligence and Relationships

Advice: Written on the back of a business card

Fortune Cookies: Small secrets on how to make a fortune

Also in the proBookmark™ Series

Daily Goals Journal:
Achieving your goals through daily action

Night Mind: Capturing the wisdom of your sleeping mind

Personal Investment Journal:
Making the right decisions for your investments

Mud & Obstacle Race Logbook

"The miracle isn't that I finished. The miracle is that I had the courage to start."

John Bingham

Obstacle races and mud runs are a virus that is spreading across the country and around the world. They awaken in people the primal spirit of play and adventure. For the first time in years, you will experience an unbounded thrill of getting out into nature to play, to run, to crawl in the mud, and to do everything that has been bread out of you as an adult.

Obstacle and mud races are mobbed by thousands of people every weekend because everyone needs a new outlet for their inner child and inner athlete.

Getting through the fear of registering for a run is the first step. Then comes the fear of showing up at the starting line. And the fear of leaping into intimidating and potentially dangerous obstacles. At the finish line, all that remains is the fear that you won't be able to do this again next weekend.

Those who finish a race are boiling over with excitement and pride in what they have accomplished.

Welcome to the family of obstacle racers and mud runners. Everyone can join. You just have to laugh at your fears and jump in.

Your Race Log

This logbook will give you performance tips and motivational messages. You will become a coauthor by contributing your own experiences on the race log sheets. Capture the joy of your race while it is still fresh in your mind. Write what is meaningful to you. Create a record that you can boast about when you are old. Paint a picture that will inspire your children to live life to the fullest.

Your inspiration is on the other side of your fears,
Roger Smith

MUD & OBSTACLE RACE LOGBOOK

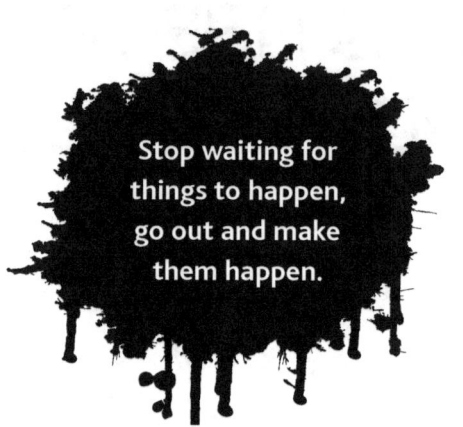

Stop waiting for things to happen, go out and make them happen.

 Racing Tip:
Chin-ups build the muscles you need to climb walls and ropes. Do these at least twice a week.

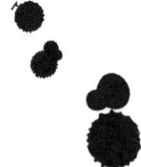

MUD & OBSTACLE RACE LOGBOOK

Race Name:	
Bib #:	Date:
Rating: ☆☆☆☆☆	Difficulty: 💀💀💀💀💀
Location:	Wave Start Time:
Race Length:	Num Obstacles:
My Run Time:	Partner/Team:
Favorite Obstacles:	
Strengths & Weaknesses:	
New Friends: (Name, Email, Facebook, Twitter)	
Race Comments: (Course, Performance, Party, Injury)	

Pre-Race Training

Sun:	Mon:
Tues:	Wed:
Thurs:	Fri:
Pre-Race Nutrition:	
Goals for the Next Race:	

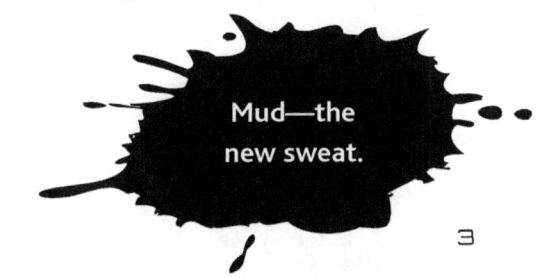

Mud—the new sweat.

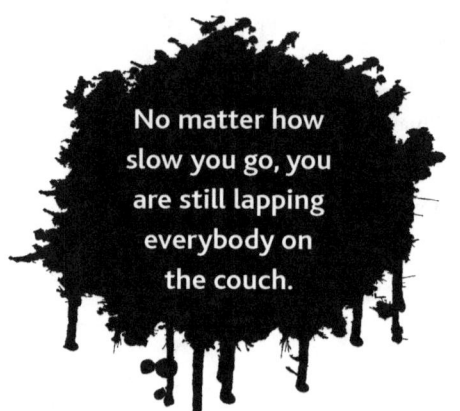

> No matter how slow you go, you are still lapping everybody on the couch.

 Racing Tip:
Good rope climbing is all in the feet. Learn the J-hook or S-wrap from Camp Rhino YouTube videos.

MUD & OBSTACLE RACE LOGBOOK

Race Name:	
Bib #:	Date:
Rating: ☆☆☆☆☆	Difficulty: 💀💀💀💀💀
Location:	Wave Start Time:
Race Length:	Num Obstacles:
My Run Time:	Partner/Team:

Favorite Obstacles:

Strengths & Weaknesses:

New Friends: (Name, Email, Facebook, Twitter)

Race Comments: (Course, Performance, Party, Injury)

Pre-Race Training

Sun:	Mon:
Tues:	Wed:
Thurs:	Fri:

Pre-Race Nutrition:

Goals for the Next Race:

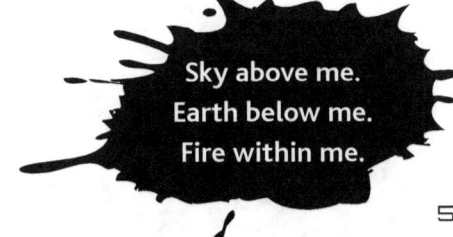

Sky above me.
Earth below me.
Fire within me.

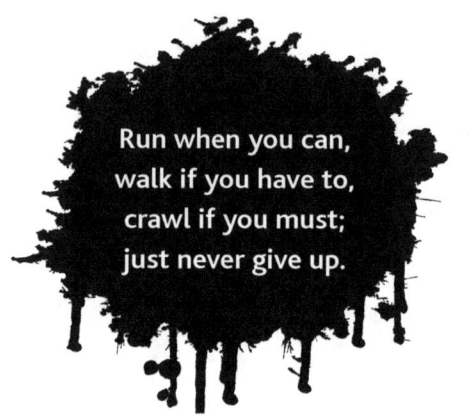

Run when you can,
walk if you have to,
crawl if you must;
just never give up.

 Racing Tip:
When you climb a tall wall, hook one heel on the top to help pull yourself over.

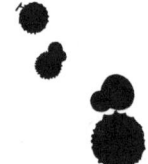

MUD & OBSTACLE RACE LOGBOOK

Race Name:	
Bib #:	Date:
Rating: ☆☆☆☆☆	Difficulty: 💀💀💀💀💀
Location:	Wave Start Time:
Race Length:	Num Obstacles:
My Run Time:	Partner/Team:

Favorite Obstacles:

Strengths & Weaknesses:

New Friends: (Name, Email, Facebook, Twitter)

Race Comments: (Course, Performance, Party, Injury)

Pre-Race Training

Sun:	Mon:
Tues:	Wed:
Thurs:	Fri:

Pre-Race Nutrition:

Goals for the Next Race:

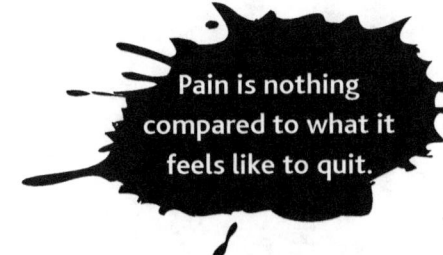

Pain is nothing compared to what it feels like to quit.

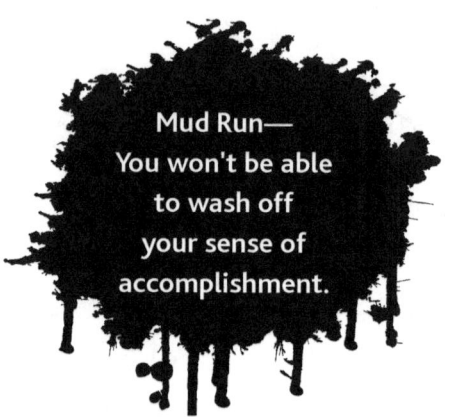

Mud Run—
You won't be able to wash off your sense of accomplishment.

 Racing Tip:
Keep a bend in your arms when doing monkey bars. Fully extended arms have less strength and are slower.

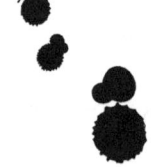

Race Name:	
Bib #:	Date:
Rating: ☆☆☆☆☆	Difficulty: 💀💀💀💀💀
Location:	Wave Start Time:
Race Length:	Num Obstacles:
My Run Time:	Partner/Team:

Favorite Obstacles:

Strengths & Weaknesses:

New Friends: (Name, Email, Facebook, Twitter)

Race Comments: (Course, Performance, Party, Injury)

Pre-Race Training

Sun:	Mon:
Tues:	Wed:
Thurs:	Fri:

Pre-Race Nutrition:

Goals for the Next Race:

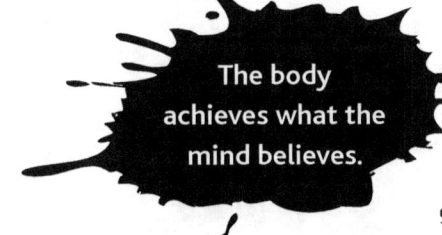

The body achieves what the mind believes.

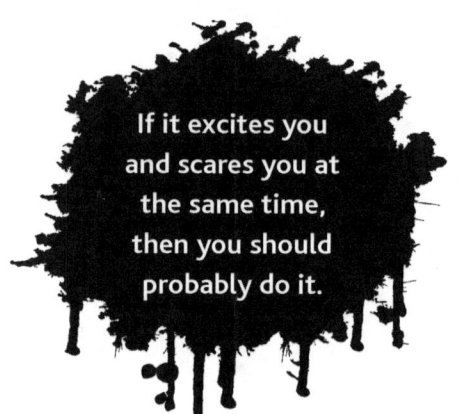

If it excites you and scares you at the same time, then you should probably do it.

 Racing Tip:
When you jump down from an obstacle, land on both feet to avoid ankle injury.

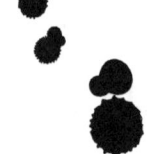

MUD & OBSTACLE RACE LOGBOOK

Race Name:	
Bib #:	Date:
Rating: ☆☆☆☆☆	Difficulty: 💀💀💀💀💀
Location:	Wave Start Time:
Race Length:	Num Obstacles:
My Run Time:	Partner/Team:
Favorite Obstacles:	
Strengths & Weaknesses:	
New Friends: (Name, Email, Facebook, Twitter)	
Race Comments: (Course, Performance, Party, Injury)	

Pre-Race Training

Sun:	Mon:
Tues:	Wed:
Thurs:	Fri:
Pre-Race Nutrition:	
Goals for the Next Race:	

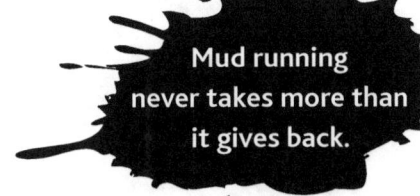

Mud running never takes more than it gives back.

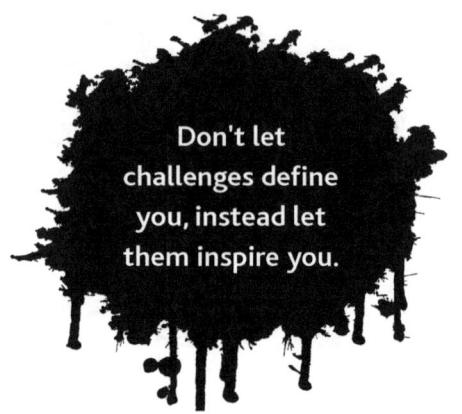

Don't let challenges define you, instead let them inspire you.

 Racing Tip:
At the beginning, run faster than your road race pace. You can slow down after a couple of obstacles.

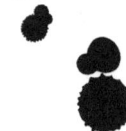

Race Name:	
Bib #:	Date:
Rating: ☆☆☆☆☆	Difficulty: 💀💀💀💀💀
Location:	Wave Start Time:
Race Length:	Num Obstacles:
My Run Time:	Partner/Team:

Favorite Obstacles:

Strengths & Weaknesses:

New Friends: (Name, Email, Facebook, Twitter)

Race Comments: (Course, Performance, Party, Injury)

Pre-Race Training

Sun:	Mon:
Tues:	Wed:
Thurs:	Fri:

Pre-Race Nutrition:

Goals for the Next Race:

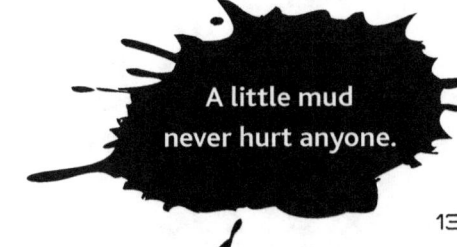

A little mud never hurt anyone.

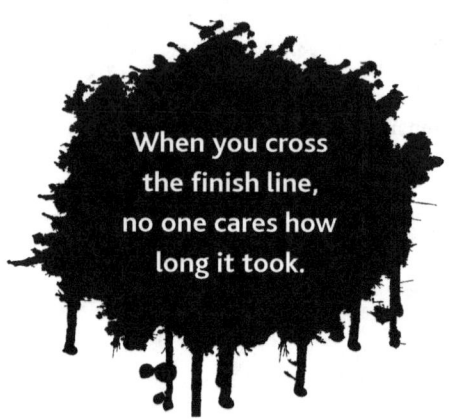

When you cross the finish line, no one cares how long it took.

Racing Tip:
Use High Intensity Interval Training to build muscle and cardio at the same time.

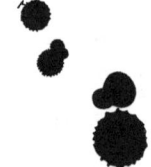

MUD & OBSTACLE RACE LOGBOOK

Race Name:	
Bib #:	Date:
Rating: ☆☆☆☆☆	Difficulty: 😈😈😈😈😈
Location:	Wave Start Time:
Race Length:	Num Obstacles:
My Run Time:	Partner/Team:

Favorite Obstacles:

Strengths & Weaknesses:

New Friends: (Name, Email, Facebook, Twitter)

Race Comments: (Course, Performance, Party, Injury)

Pre-Race Training

Sun:	Mon:
Tues:	Wed:
Thurs:	Fri:

Pre-Race Nutrition:

Goals for the Next Race:

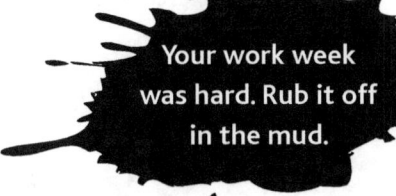

Your work week was hard. Rub it off in the mud.

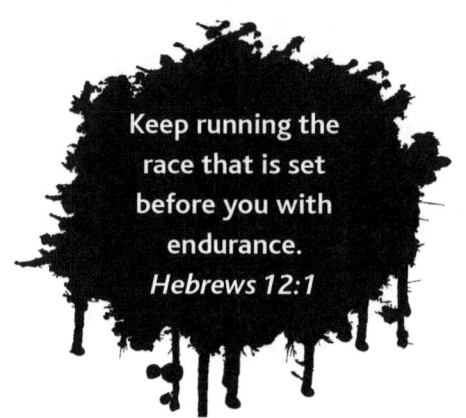

Keep running the race that is set before you with endurance.
Hebrews 12:1

Racing Tip:

Try a Tabata workout with 20 seconds of exercise, followed by 10 seconds of rest, repeated 8 times. Then rest for one minute and do it again with a different exercise.

MUD & OBSTACLE RACE LOGBOOK

Race Name:	
Bib #:	Date:
Rating: ☆☆☆☆☆	Difficulty: 💀💀💀💀💀
Location:	Wave Start Time:
Race Length:	Num Obstacles:
My Run Time:	Partner/Team:
Favorite Obstacles:	
Strengths & Weaknesses:	
New Friends: (Name, Email, Facebook, Twitter)	
Race Comments: (Course, Performance, Party, Injury)	

Pre-Race Training

Sun:	Mon:
Tues:	Wed:
Thurs:	Fri:
Pre-Race Nutrition:	
Goals for the Next Race:	

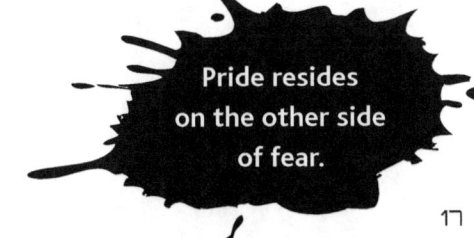

Pride resides on the other side of fear.

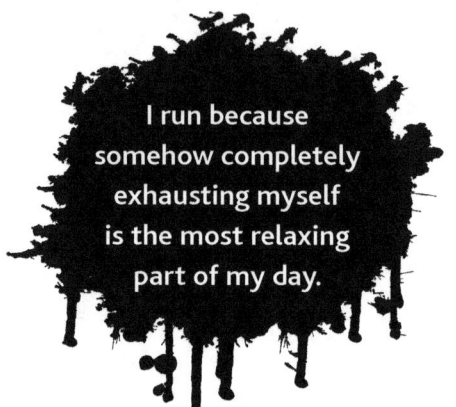

I run because somehow completely exhausting myself is the most relaxing part of my day.

 Racing Tip:
Burpees are the signature exercise of obstacle racing. Do 30 every day.

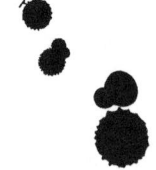

Race Name:	
Bib #:	Date:
Rating: ☆☆☆☆☆	Difficulty: 💀💀💀💀💀
Location:	Wave Start Time:
Race Length:	Num Obstacles:
My Run Time:	Partner/Team:
Favorite Obstacles:	
Strengths & Weaknesses:	
New Friends: (Name, Email, Facebook, Twitter)	
Race Comments: (Course, Performance, Party, Injury)	

Pre-Race Training

Sun:	Mon:
Tues:	Wed:
Thurs:	Fri:
Pre-Race Nutrition:	
Goals for the Next Race:	

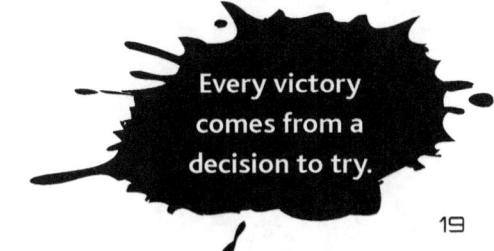

Every victory comes from a decision to try.

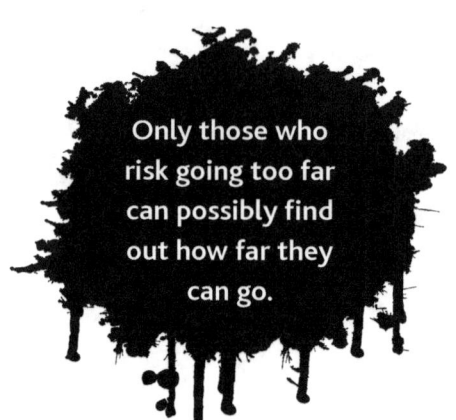

Only those who risk going too far can possibly find out how far they can go.

 Racing Tip:
Oatmeal is the perfect long-lasting, low fat, stomach filling energy food. Eat it daily for breakfast.

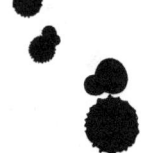

MUD & OBSTACLE RACE LOGBOOK

Race Name:	
Bib #:	Date:
Rating: ☆☆☆☆☆	Difficulty: 💀💀💀💀💀
Location:	Wave Start Time:
Race Length:	Num Obstacles:
My Run Time:	Partner/Team:
Favorite Obstacles:	

Strengths & Weaknesses:

New Friends: (Name, Email, Facebook, Twitter)

Race Comments: (Course, Performance, Party, Injury)

Pre-Race Training

Sun:	Mon:
Tues:	Wed:
Thurs:	Fri:

Pre-Race Nutrition:

Goals for the Next Race:

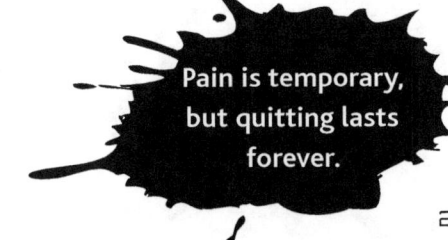

Pain is temporary, but quitting lasts forever.

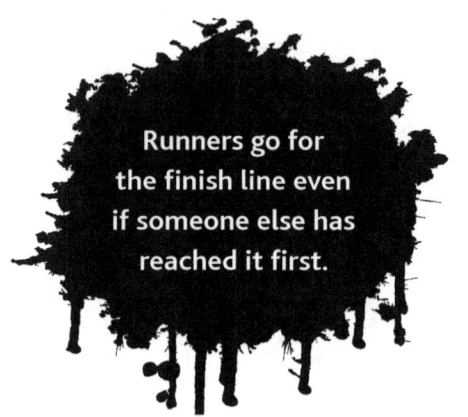

Runners go for the finish line even if someone else has reached it first.

 Racing Tip:
Make great shakes with protein powder, juice, almond milk, ground flax seed, nut butter, cinnamon, and fruit.

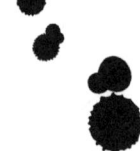

MUD & OBSTACLE RACE LOGBOOK

Race Name:	
Bib #:	Date:
Rating: ☆☆☆☆☆	Difficulty: 💀💀💀💀💀
Location:	Wave Start Time:
Race Length:	Num Obstacles:
My Run Time:	Partner/Team:

Favorite Obstacles:

Strengths & Weaknesses:

New Friends: (Name, Email, Facebook, Twitter)

Race Comments: (Course, Performance, Party, Injury)

Pre-Race Training

Sun:	Mon:
Tues:	Wed:
Thurs:	Fri:

Pre-Race Nutrition:

Goals for the Next Race:

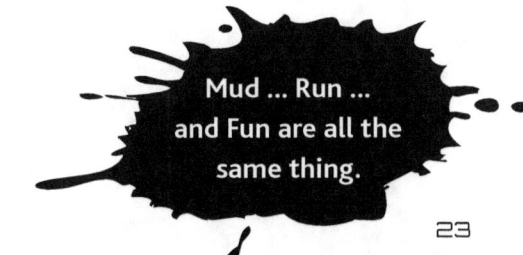

Mud ... Run ... and Fun are all the same thing.

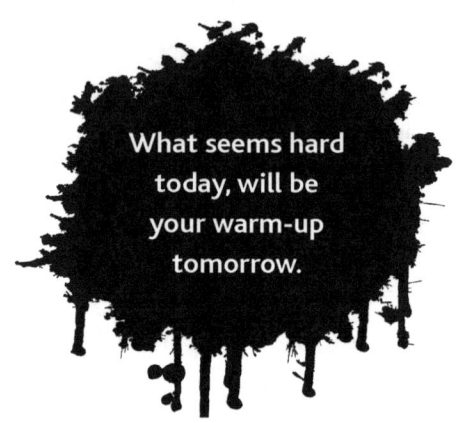

What seems hard today, will be your warm-up tomorrow.

 Racing Tip:
Do a yoga-pilates workout twice a week for flexibility and to avoid injury.

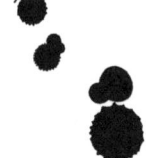

MUD & OBSTACLE RACE LOGBOOK

Race Name:	
Bib #:	Date:
Rating: ☆☆☆☆☆	Difficulty: ☠☠☠☠☠
Location:	Wave Start Time:
Race Length:	Num Obstacles:
My Run Time:	Partner/Team:
Favorite Obstacles:	
Strengths & Weaknesses:	
New Friends: (Name, Email, Facebook, Twitter)	
Race Comments: (Course, Performance, Party, Injury)	

Pre-Race Training

Sun:	Mon:
Tues:	Wed:
Thurs:	Fri:
Pre-Race Nutrition:	
Goals for the Next Race:	

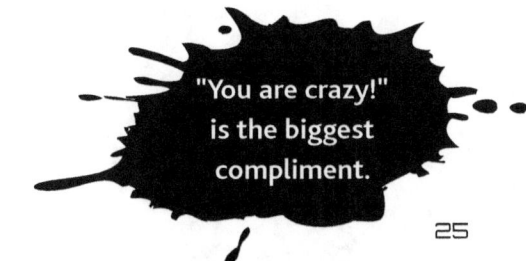

"You are crazy!" is the biggest compliment.

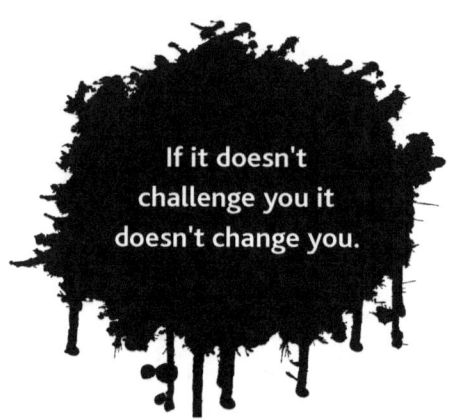

If it doesn't challenge you it doesn't change you.

 Racing Tip:
Run at least twice a week, one long and one fast.

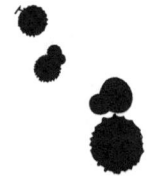

MUD & OBSTACLE RACE LOGBOOK

Race Name:	
Bib #:	Date:
Rating: ☆☆☆☆☆	Difficulty: 💀💀💀💀💀
Location:	Wave Start Time:
Race Length:	Num Obstacles:
My Run Time:	Partner/Team:
Favorite Obstacles:	
Strengths & Weaknesses:	
New Friends: (Name, Email, Facebook, Twitter)	
Race Comments: (Course, Performance, Party, Injury)	

Pre-Race Training

Sun:	Mon:
Tues:	Wed:
Thurs:	Fri:
Pre-Race Nutrition:	
Goals for the Next Race:	

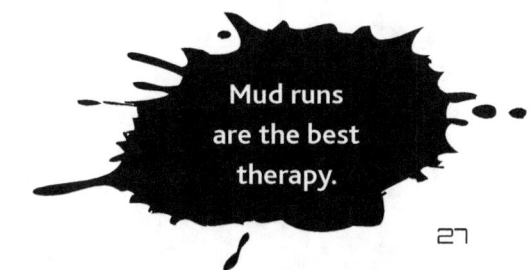

Mud runs are the best therapy.

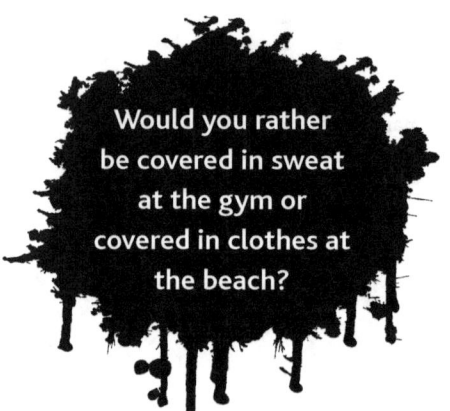

Would you rather be covered in sweat at the gym or covered in clothes at the beach?

 Racing Tip:
Rest the day before a race so your body can store energy for the big event.

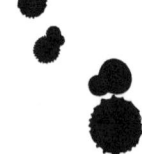

MUD & OBSTACLE RACE LOGBOOK

Race Name:	
Bib #:	Date:
Rating: ☆☆☆☆☆	Difficulty: 💀💀💀💀💀
Location:	Wave Start Time:
Race Length:	Num Obstacles:
My Run Time:	Partner/Team:

Favorite Obstacles:

Strengths & Weaknesses:

New Friends: (Name, Email, Facebook, Twitter)

Race Comments: (Course, Performance, Party, Injury)

Pre-Race Training

Sun:	Mon:
Tues:	Wed:
Thurs:	Fri:

Pre-Race Nutrition:

Goals for the Next Race:

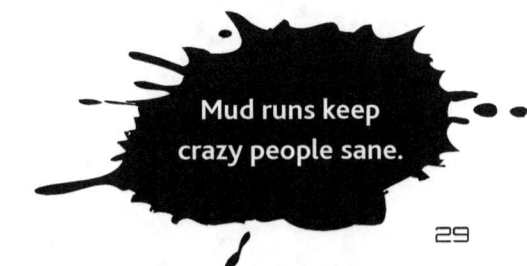

Mud runs keep crazy people sane.

29

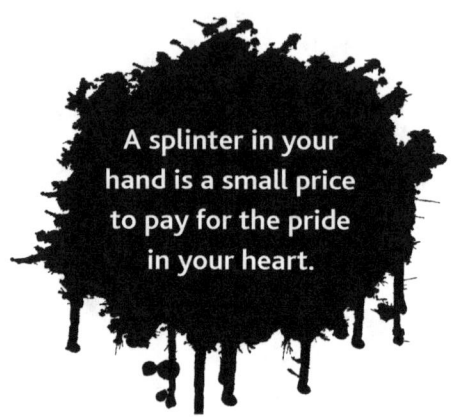

A splinter in your hand is a small price to pay for the pride in your heart.

 Racing Tip:
Twice during your work day take a five minute mental break. Meditate or walk outside.

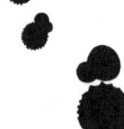

MUD & OBSTACLE RACE LOGBOOK

Race Name:	
Bib #:	Date:
Rating: ☆☆☆☆☆	Difficulty: 💀💀💀💀💀
Location:	Wave Start Time:
Race Length:	Num Obstacles:
My Run Time:	Partner/Team:
Favorite Obstacles:	

Strengths & Weaknesses:

New Friends: (Name, Email, Facebook, Twitter)

Race Comments: (Course, Performance, Party, Injury)

Pre-Race Training

Sun:	Mon:
Tues:	Wed:
Thurs:	Fri:
Pre-Race Nutrition:	

Goals for the Next Race:

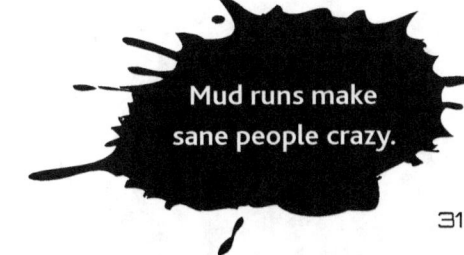

Mud runs make sane people crazy.

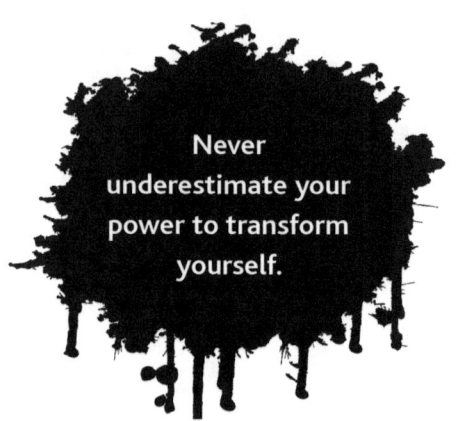

Never underestimate your power to transform yourself.

 Racing Tip:
Choose to eat foods with just one ingredient, like chicken, vegetables, fruits, and nuts.

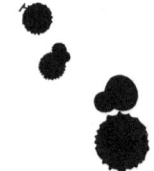

Race Name:	
Bib #:	Date:
Rating: ☆☆☆☆☆	Difficulty: 💀💀💀💀💀
Location:	Wave Start Time:
Race Length:	Num Obstacles:
My Run Time:	Partner/Team:
Favorite Obstacles:	
Strengths & Weaknesses:	
New Friends: (Name, Email, Facebook, Twitter)	
Race Comments: (Course, Performance, Party, Injury)	

Pre-Race Training

Sun:	Mon:
Tues:	Wed:
Thurs:	Fri:
Pre-Race Nutrition:	
Goals for the Next Race:	

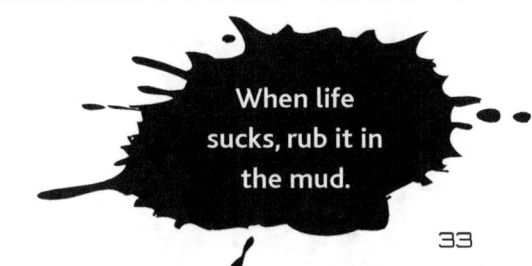

When life sucks, rub it in the mud.

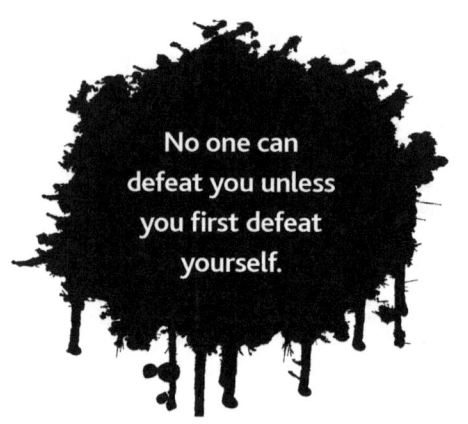

> No one can defeat you unless you first defeat yourself.

 Racing Tip:
Hydrate before a race at 2 days, 2 hours, 2 minutes, and 2 miles into the race.

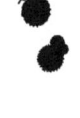

MUD & OBSTACLE RACE LOGBOOK

Race Name:	
Bib #:	Date:
Rating: ☆☆☆☆☆	Difficulty: 💀💀💀💀💀
Location:	Wave Start Time:
Race Length:	Num Obstacles:
My Run Time:	Partner/Team:
Favorite Obstacles:	
Strengths & Weaknesses:	
New Friends: (Name, Email, Facebook, Twitter)	
Race Comments: (Course, Performance, Party, Injury)	

Pre-Race Training

Sun:	Mon:
Tues:	Wed:
Thurs:	Fri:
Pre-Race Nutrition:	
Goals for the Next Race:	

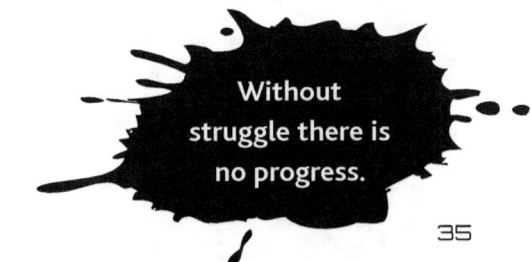

Without struggle there is no progress.

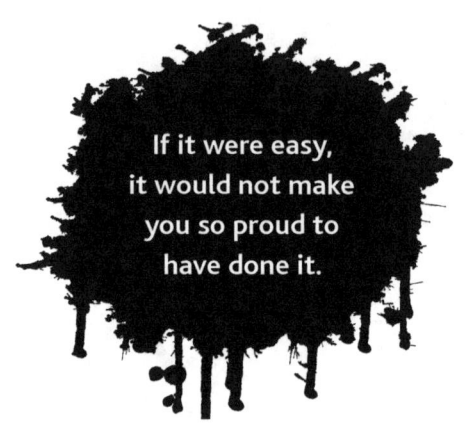

If it were easy,
it would not make
you so proud to
have done it.

 Racing Tip:
Apply sun block and SPF lip balm before you leave your car.

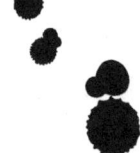

MUD & OBSTACLE RACE LOGBOOK

Race Name:	
Bib #:	Date:
Rating: ☆☆☆☆☆	Difficulty: 💀💀💀💀💀
Location:	Wave Start Time:
Race Length:	Num Obstacles:
My Run Time:	Partner/Team:
Favorite Obstacles:	

Strengths & Weaknesses:

New Friends: (Name, Email, Facebook, Twitter)

Race Comments: (Course, Performance, Party, Injury)

Pre-Race Training

Sun:	Mon:
Tues:	Wed:
Thurs:	Fri:
Pre-Race Nutrition:	

Goals for the Next Race:

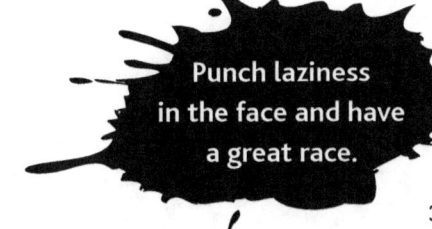

Punch laziness in the face and have a great race.

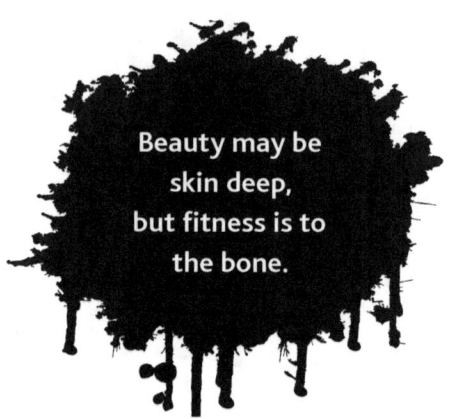

Beauty may be skin deep, but fitness is to the bone.

 Racing Tip:
All obstacles are optional. Do not be macho if the obstacle is dangerous for you.

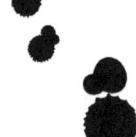

Race Name:	
Bib #:	Date:
Rating: ☆☆☆☆☆	Difficulty: 💀💀💀💀💀
Location:	Wave Start Time:
Race Length:	Num Obstacles:
My Run Time:	Partner/Team:
Favorite Obstacles:	
Strengths & Weaknesses:	
New Friends: (Name, Email, Facebook, Twitter)	
Race Comments: (Course, Performance, Party, Injury)	

Pre-Race Training

Sun:	Mon:
Tues:	Wed:
Thurs:	Fri:
Pre-Race Nutrition:	
Goals for the Next Race:	

Breathe in the future, breathe out the past.

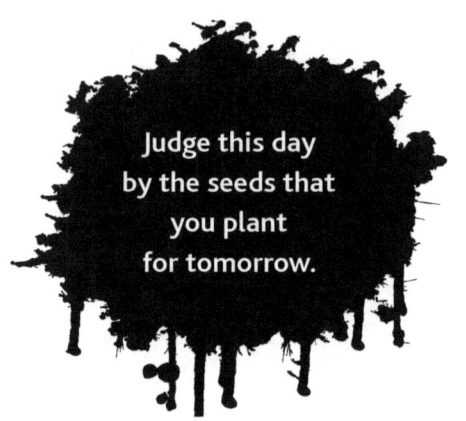

Judge this day
by the seeds that
you plant
for tomorrow.

 Racing Tip:
Like the race Facebook page.
You will learn important tips
and get discounts.

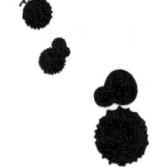

Race Name:	
Bib #:	Date:
Rating: ☆☆☆☆☆	Difficulty: 💀💀💀💀💀
Location:	Wave Start Time:
Race Length:	Num Obstacles:
My Run Time:	Partner/Team:

Favorite Obstacles:

Strengths & Weaknesses:

New Friends: (Name, Email, Facebook, Twitter)

Race Comments: (Course, Performance, Party, Injury)

Pre-Race Training

Sun:	Mon:
Tues:	Wed:
Thurs:	Fri:

Pre-Race Nutrition:

Goals for the Next Race:

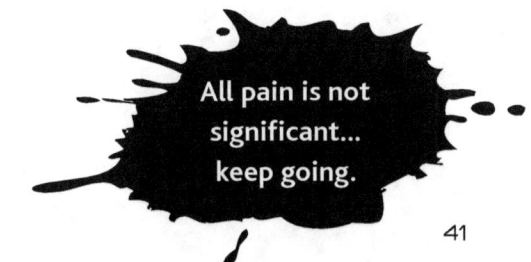

All pain is not significant... keep going.

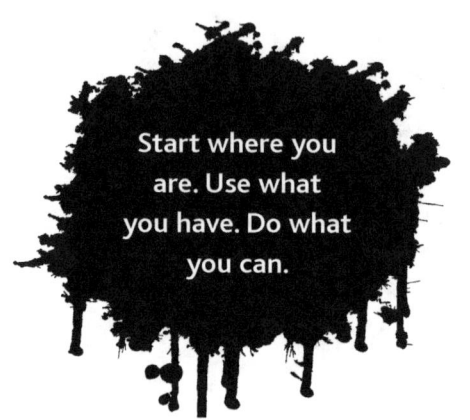

> Start where you are. Use what you have. Do what you can.

 Racing Tip:
Make new friends at the race. Everyone is excited, a little nervous, and ready to talk about the experience.

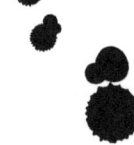

MUD & OBSTACLE RACE LOGBOOK

Race Name:	
Bib #:	Date:
Rating: ☆☆☆☆☆	Difficulty: 💀💀💀💀💀
Location:	Wave Start Time:
Race Length:	Num Obstacles:
My Run Time:	Partner/Team:
Favorite Obstacles:	
Strengths & Weaknesses:	
New Friends: (Name, Email, Facebook, Twitter)	
Race Comments: (Course, Performance, Party, Injury)	

Pre-Race Training

Sun:	Mon:
Tues:	Wed:
Thurs:	Fri:
Pre-Race Nutrition:	
Goals for the Next Race:	

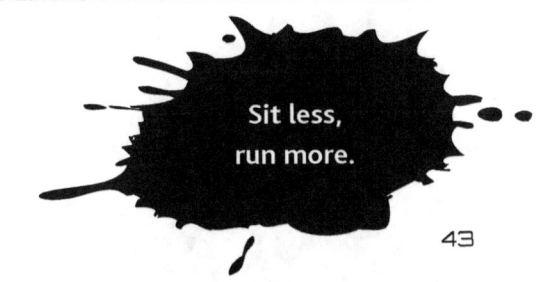

Sit less, run more.

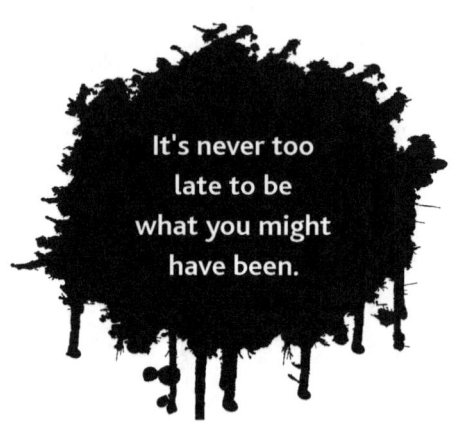

It's never too
late to be
what you might
have been.

 Racing Tip:

Join a team or make a team. Races are more fun in a group. Check out MudRunFun.com to get started.

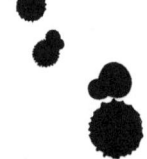

Race Name:	
Bib #:	Date:
Rating: ☆☆☆☆☆	Difficulty: 💀💀💀💀💀
Location:	Wave Start Time:
Race Length:	Num Obstacles:
My Run Time:	Partner/Team:

Favorite Obstacles:

Strengths & Weaknesses:

New Friends: (Name, Email, Facebook, Twitter)

Race Comments: (Course, Performance, Party, Injury)

Pre-Race Training

Sun:	Mon:
Tues:	Wed:
Thurs:	Fri:

Pre-Race Nutrition:

Goals for the Next Race:

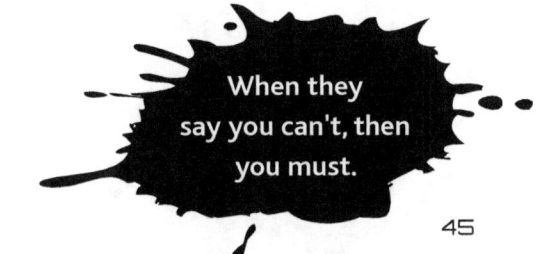

When they say you can't, then you must.

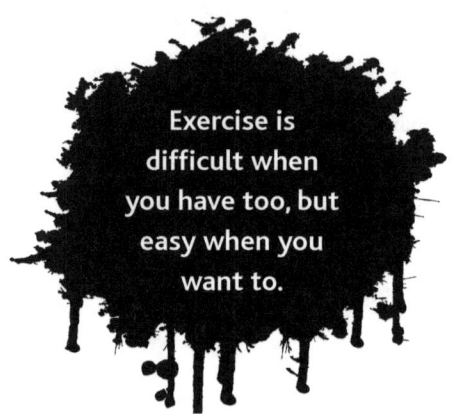

Exercise is difficult when you have too, but easy when you want to.

 Racing Tip:
Wear compression sleeves on your legs and arms to protect against cuts and scrapes.

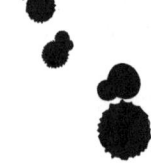

MUD & OBSTACLE RACE LOGBOOK

Race Name:	
Bib #:	Date:
Rating: ☆☆☆☆☆	Difficulty: 💀💀💀💀💀
Location:	Wave Start Time:
Race Length:	Num Obstacles:
My Run Time:	Partner/Team:
Favorite Obstacles:	
Strengths & Weaknesses:	
New Friends: (Name, Email, Facebook, Twitter)	
Race Comments: (Course, Performance, Party, Injury)	

Pre-Race Training

Sun:	Mon:
Tues:	Wed:
Thurs:	Fri:
Pre-Race Nutrition:	
Goals for the Next Race:	

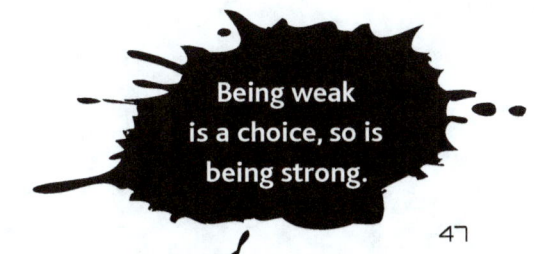

Being weak is a choice, so is being strong.

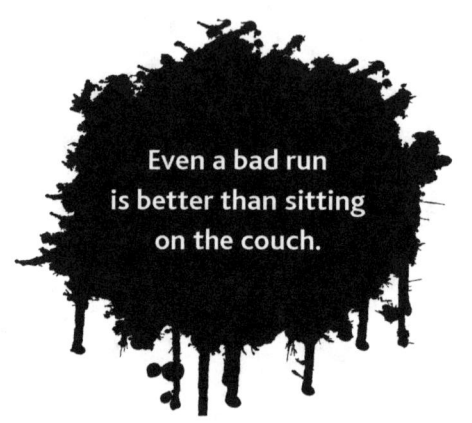

Even a bad run is better than sitting on the couch.

 Racing Tip:
Most gloves are terrible for wet obstacles. Go barehanded.

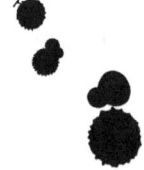

MUD & OBSTACLE RACE LOGBOOK

Race Name:	
Bib #:	Date:
Rating: ☆☆☆☆☆	Difficulty: 💀💀💀💀💀
Location:	Wave Start Time:
Race Length:	Num Obstacles:
My Run Time:	Partner/Team:
Favorite Obstacles:	
Strengths & Weaknesses:	
New Friends: (Name, Email, Facebook, Twitter)	
Race Comments: (Course, Performance, Party, Injury)	

Pre-Race Training

Sun:	Mon:
Tues:	Wed:
Thurs:	Fri:
Pre-Race Nutrition:	
Goals for the Next Race:	

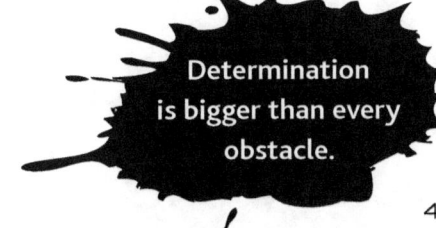

Determination is bigger than every obstacle.

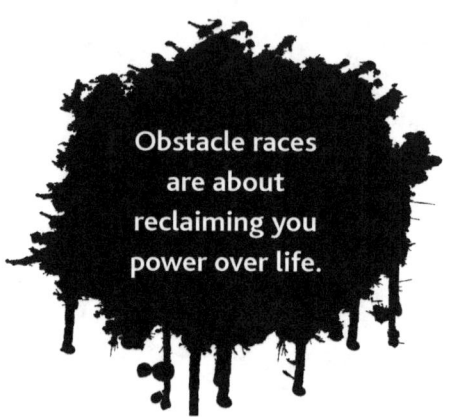

Obstacle races are about reclaiming you power over life.

 Racing Tip:
Race in good running shoes, not worn out yard shoes.

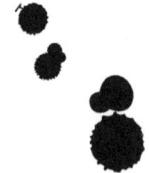

MUD & OBSTACLE RACE LOGBOOK

Race Name:	
Bib #:	Date:
Rating: ☆☆☆☆☆	Difficulty: 💀💀💀💀💀
Location:	Wave Start Time:
Race Length:	Num Obstacles:
My Run Time:	Partner/Team:
Favorite Obstacles:	
Strengths & Weaknesses:	
New Friends: (Name, Email, Facebook, Twitter)	
Race Comments: (Course, Performance, Party, Injury)	

Pre-Race Training

Sun:	Mon:
Tues:	Wed:
Thurs:	Fri:
Pre-Race Nutrition:	
Goals for the Next Race:	

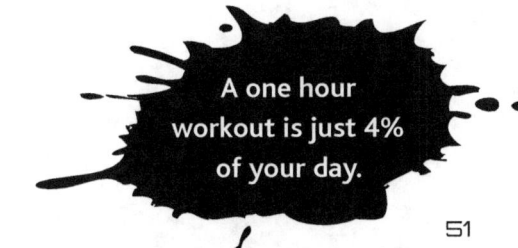

A one hour workout is just 4% of your day.

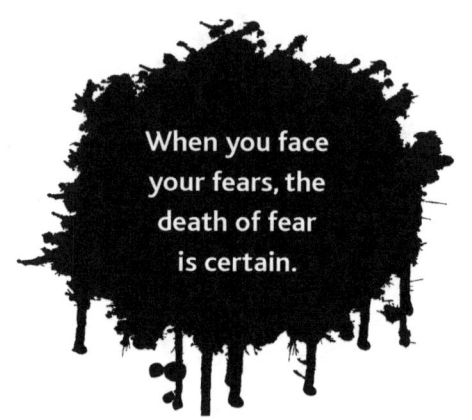

When you face your fears, the death of fear is certain.

 Racing Tip:
Machine wash your shoes after the race. It won't hurt them.

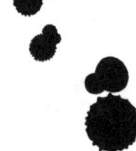

Race Name:	
Bib #:	Date:
Rating: ☆☆☆☆☆	Difficulty: 💀💀💀💀💀
Location:	Wave Start Time:
Race Length:	Num Obstacles:
My Run Time:	Partner/Team:

Favorite Obstacles:

Strengths & Weaknesses:

New Friends: (Name, Email, Facebook, Twitter)

Race Comments: (Course, Performance, Party, Injury)

Pre-Race Training

Sun:	Mon:
Tues:	Wed:
Thurs:	Fri:

Pre-Race Nutrition:

Goals for the Next Race:

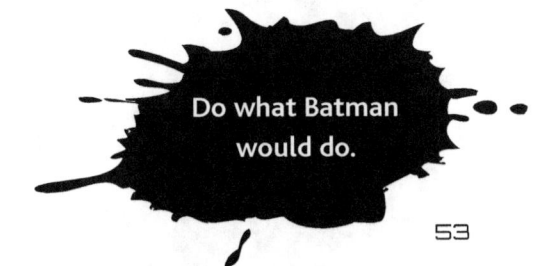

Do what Batman would do.

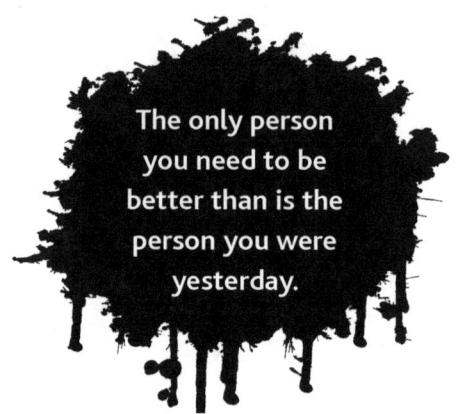

The only person you need to be better than is the person you were yesterday.

 Racing Tip:
Do 10 minutes of exercise every morning to jump start your muscles and metabolism.

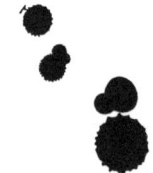

MUD & OBSTACLE RACE LOGBOOK

Race Name:	
Bib #:	Date:
Rating: ☆☆☆☆☆	Difficulty: ☠☠☠☠☠
Location:	Wave Start Time:
Race Length:	Num Obstacles:
My Run Time:	Partner/Team:
Favorite Obstacles:	
Strengths & Weaknesses:	
New Friends: (Name, Email, Facebook, Twitter)	
Race Comments: (Course, Performance, Party, Injury)	

Pre-Race Training

Sun:	Mon:
Tues:	Wed:
Thurs:	Fri:
Pre-Race Nutrition:	
Goals for the Next Race:	

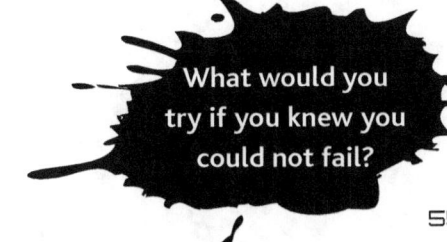

What would you try if you knew you could not fail?

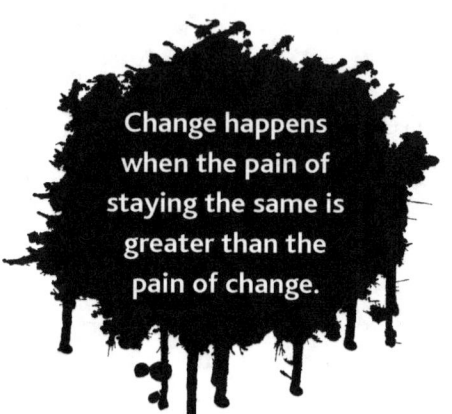

Change happens when the pain of staying the same is greater than the pain of change.

 Racing Tip:
Eat salad at least twice a week. You need the water, fiber, and nutrients.

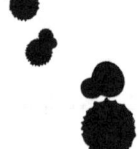

Race Name:	
Bib #:	Date:
Rating: ☆☆☆☆☆	Difficulty: ☠☠☠☠☠
Location:	Wave Start Time:
Race Length:	Num Obstacles:
My Run Time:	Partner/Team:
Favorite Obstacles:	
Strengths & Weaknesses:	
New Friends: (Name, Email, Facebook, Twitter)	
Race Comments: (Course, Performance, Party, Injury)	

Pre-Race Training

Sun:	Mon:
Tues:	Wed:
Thurs:	Fri:
Pre-Race Nutrition:	
Goals for the Next Race:	

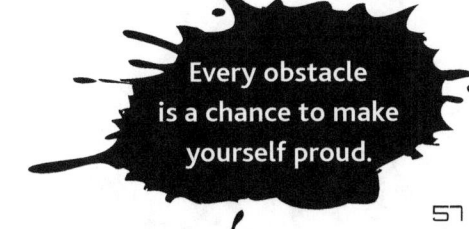

Every obstacle is a chance to make yourself proud.

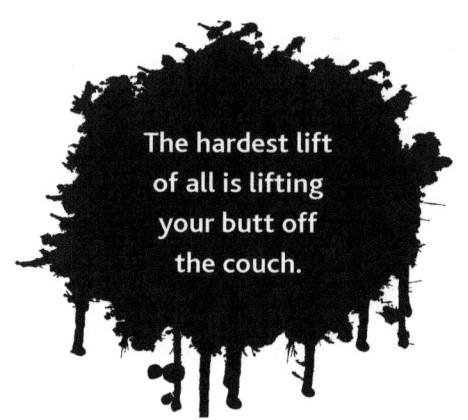

The hardest lift of all is lifting your butt off the couch.

 Racing Tip:
Smile when you are exhausted, it will give you more energy.

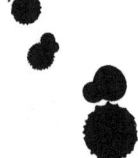

MUD & OBSTACLE RACE LOGBOOK

Race Name:	
Bib #:	Date:
Rating: ☆☆☆☆☆	Difficulty: 💀💀💀💀💀
Location:	Wave Start Time:
Race Length:	Num Obstacles:
My Run Time:	Partner/Team:
Favorite Obstacles:	

Strengths & Weaknesses:

New Friends: (Name, Email, Facebook, Twitter)

Race Comments: (Course, Performance, Party, Injury)

Pre-Race Training

Sun:	Mon:
Tues:	Wed:
Thurs:	Fri:
Pre-Race Nutrition:	

Goals for the Next Race:

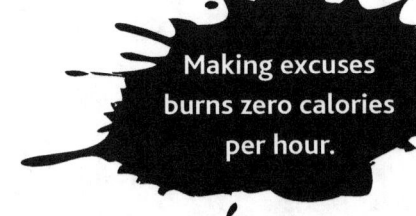

Making excuses burns zero calories per hour.

59

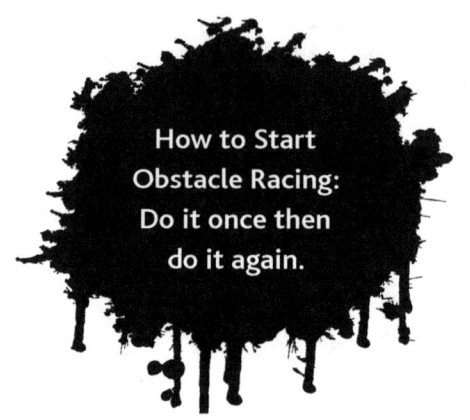

How to Start
Obstacle Racing:
Do it once then
do it again.

 Racing Tip:
Laugh when you make a mistake, it chases away the self-criticism.

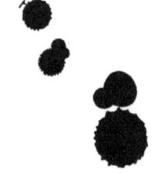

MUD & OBSTACLE RACE LOGBOOK

Race Name:	
Bib #:	Date:
Rating: ☆☆☆☆☆	Difficulty: 💀💀💀💀💀
Location:	Wave Start Time:
Race Length:	Num Obstacles:
My Run Time:	Partner/Team:

Favorite Obstacles:

Strengths & Weaknesses:

New Friends: (Name, Email, Facebook, Twitter)

Race Comments: (Course, Performance, Party, Injury)

Pre-Race Training

Sun:	Mon:
Tues:	Wed:
Thurs:	Fri:

Pre-Race Nutrition:

Goals for the Next Race:

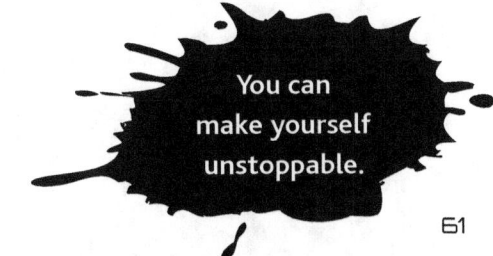

You can make yourself unstoppable.

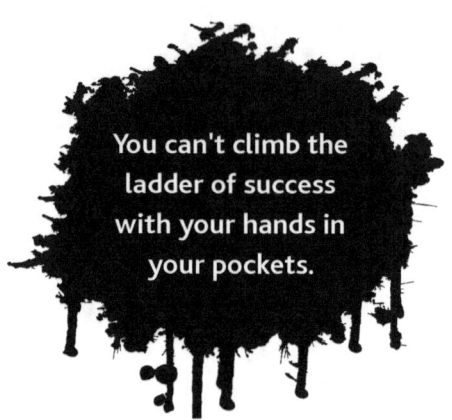

You can't climb the ladder of success with your hands in your pockets.

 Racing Tip:
A one hour work out is just 4% of each day, you can afford the time.

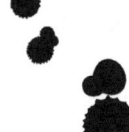

Race Name:	
Bib #:	Date:
Rating: ☆☆☆☆☆	Difficulty: 💀💀💀💀💀
Location:	Wave Start Time:
Race Length:	Num Obstacles:
My Run Time:	Partner/Team:
Favorite Obstacles:	
Strengths & Weaknesses:	
New Friends: (Name, Email, Facebook, Twitter)	
Race Comments: (Course, Performance, Party, Injury)	

Pre-Race Training

Sun:	Mon:
Tues:	Wed:
Thurs:	Fri:
Pre-Race Nutrition:	
Goals for the Next Race:	

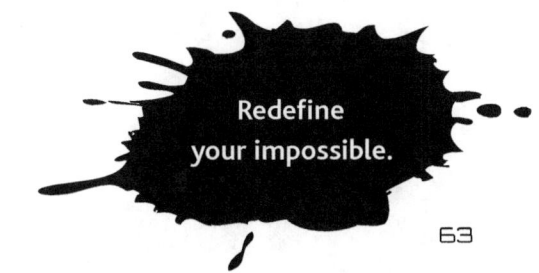

Redefine your impossible.

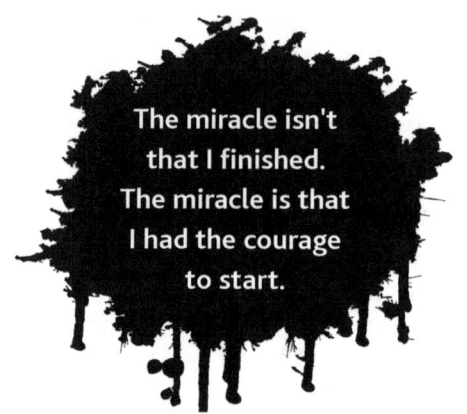

The miracle isn't that I finished. The miracle is that I had the courage to start.

 Racing Tip:
Look before you leap into an obstacle.

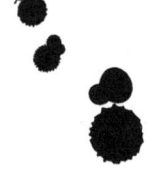

MUD & OBSTACLE RACE LOGBOOK

Race Name:	
Bib #:	Date:
Rating: ☆☆☆☆☆	Difficulty: 💀💀💀💀💀
Location:	Wave Start Time:
Race Length:	Num Obstacles:
My Run Time:	Partner/Team:
Favorite Obstacles:	

Strengths & Weaknesses:

New Friends: (Name, Email, Facebook, Twitter)

Race Comments: (Course, Performance, Party, Injury)

Pre-Race Training

Sun:	Mon:
Tues:	Wed:
Thurs:	Fri:
Pre-Race Nutrition:	

Goals for the Next Race:

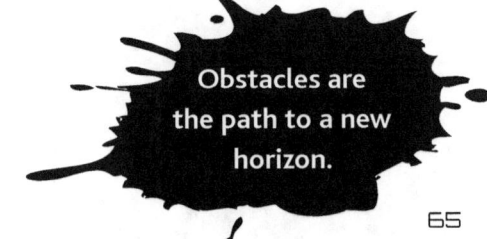

Obstacles are the path to a new horizon.

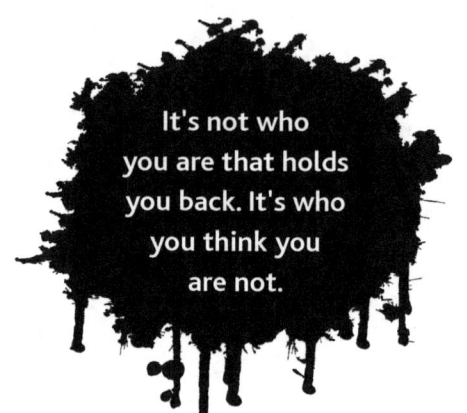

It's not who you are that holds you back. It's who you think you are not.

 Racing Tip:
Do yoga the day after a race. Your muscles and joints will love you for it. It is a fantastic recovery workout.

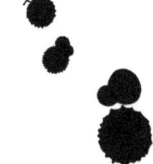

MUD & OBSTACLE RACE LOGBOOK

Race Name:	
Bib #:	Date:
Rating: ☆☆☆☆☆	Difficulty: 💀💀💀💀💀
Location:	Wave Start Time:
Race Length:	Num Obstacles:
My Run Time:	Partner/Team:

Favorite Obstacles:

Strengths & Weaknesses:

New Friends: (Name, Email, Facebook, Twitter)

Race Comments: (Course, Performance, Party, Injury)

Pre-Race Training

Sun:	Mon:
Tues:	Wed:
Thurs:	Fri:

Pre-Race Nutrition:

Goals for the Next Race:

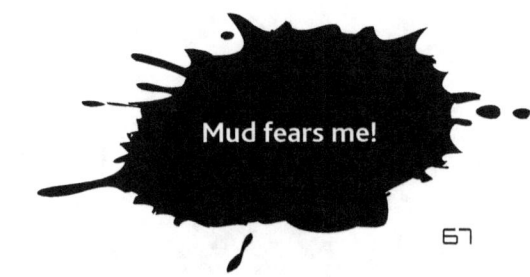
Mud fears me!

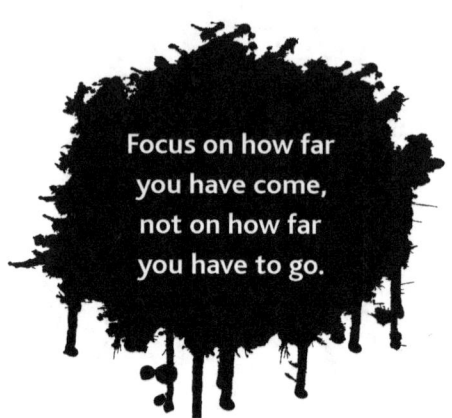

Focus on how far you have come, not on how far you have to go.

 Racing Tip:
Watch other people do the obstacles to learn technique and build confidence.

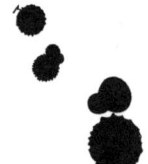

MUD & OBSTACLE RACE LOGBOOK

Race Name:	
Bib #:	Date:
Rating: ☆☆☆☆☆	Difficulty: 💀💀💀💀💀
Location:	Wave Start Time:
Race Length:	Num Obstacles:
My Run Time:	Partner/Team:
Favorite Obstacles:	
Strengths & Weaknesses:	
New Friends: (Name, Email, Facebook, Twitter)	
Race Comments: (Course, Performance, Party, Injury)	

Pre-Race Training

Sun:	Mon:
Tues:	Wed:
Thurs:	Fri:
Pre-Race Nutrition:	
Goals for the Next Race:	

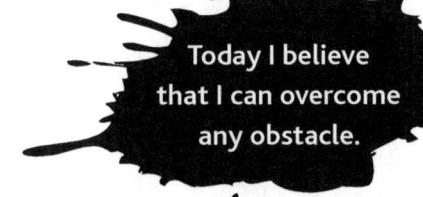

Today I believe that I can overcome any obstacle.

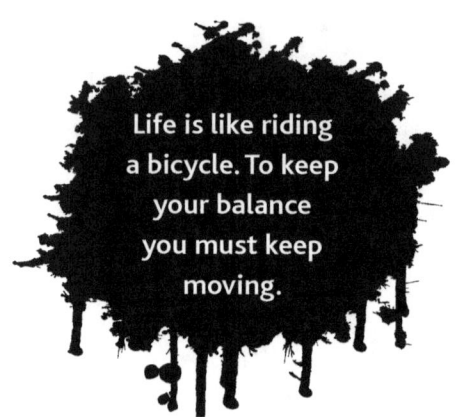

Life is like riding a bicycle. To keep your balance you must keep moving.

 Racing Tip:
Dry your hands on grass or leaves as you approach monkey bars or ropes.

MUD & OBSTACLE RACE LOGBOOK

Race Name:	
Bib #:	Date:
Rating: ☆☆☆☆☆	Difficulty: 💀💀💀💀💀
Location:	Wave Start Time:
Race Length:	Num Obstacles:
My Run Time:	Partner/Team:
Favorite Obstacles:	
Strengths & Weaknesses:	
New Friends: (Name, Email, Facebook, Twitter)	
Race Comments: (Course, Performance, Party, Injury)	

Pre-Race Training

Sun:	Mon:
Tues:	Wed:
Thurs:	Fri:
Pre-Race Nutrition:	
Goals for the Next Race:	

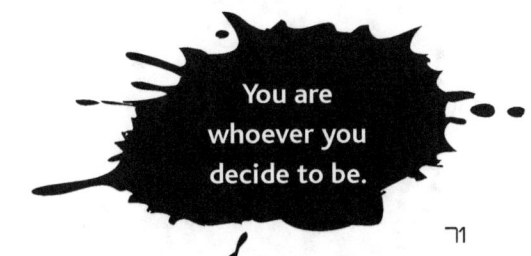

You are whoever you decide to be.

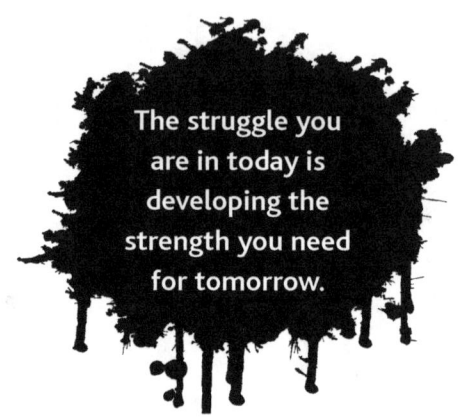

The struggle you are in today is developing the strength you need for tomorrow.

 Racing Tip:
Cover your face when you run through electric shock. The shock is 90% psychological and 10% physical.

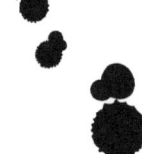

Race Name:	
Bib #:	Date:
Rating: ☆☆☆☆☆	Difficulty: 💀💀💀💀💀
Location:	Wave Start Time:
Race Length:	Num Obstacles:
My Run Time:	Partner/Team:
Favorite Obstacles:	
Strengths & Weaknesses:	
New Friends: (Name, Email, Facebook, Twitter)	
Race Comments: (Course, Performance, Party, Injury)	

Pre-Race Training

Sun:	Mon:
Tues:	Wed:
Thurs:	Fri:
Pre-Race Nutrition:	
Goals for the Next Race:	

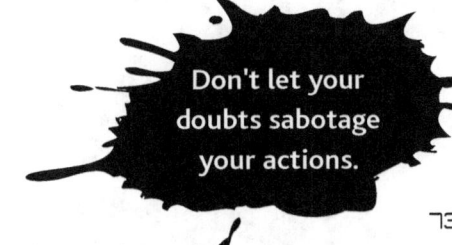

Don't let your doubts sabotage your actions.

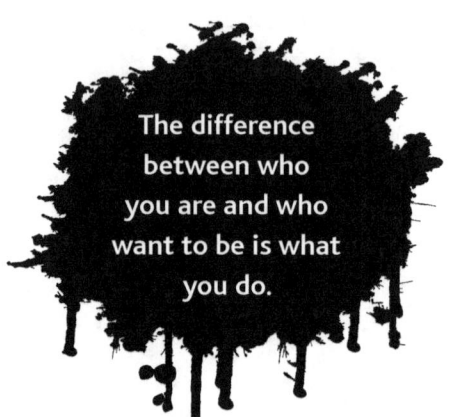

The difference between who you are and who want to be is what you do.

 Racing Tip:
Parkour can teach you to run up a 14' wall. Check YouTube for instructions.

MUD & OBSTACLE RACE LOGBOOK

Race Name:	
Bib #:	Date:
Rating: ☆☆☆☆☆	Difficulty: 💀💀💀💀💀
Location:	Wave Start Time:
Race Length:	Num Obstacles:
My Run Time:	Partner/Team:

Favorite Obstacles:

Strengths & Weaknesses:

New Friends: (Name, Email, Facebook, Twitter)

Race Comments: (Course, Performance, Party, Injury)

Pre-Race Training

Sun:	Mon:
Tues:	Wed:
Thurs:	Fri:

Pre-Race Nutrition:

Goals for the Next Race:

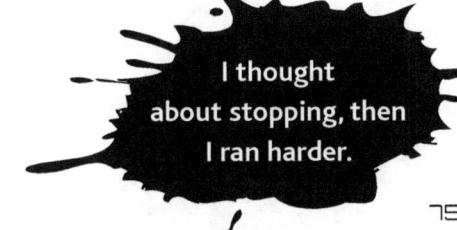

I thought about stopping, then I ran harder.

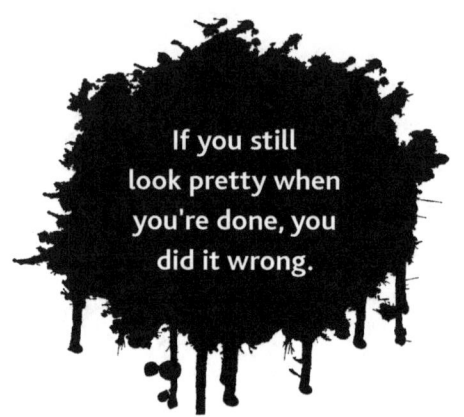

If you still look pretty when you're done, you did it wrong.

 Racing Tip:
Don't duct tape your shoes.
It does not keep the water out
and you lose your running traction.

MUD & OBSTACLE RACE LOGBOOK

Race Name:	
Bib #:	Date:
Rating: ☆☆☆☆☆	Difficulty: 💀💀💀💀💀
Location:	Wave Start Time:
Race Length:	Num Obstacles:
My Run Time:	Partner/Team:
Favorite Obstacles:	

Strengths & Weaknesses:

New Friends: (Name, Email, Facebook, Twitter)

Race Comments: (Course, Performance, Party, Injury)

Pre-Race Training

Sun:	Mon:
Tues:	Wed:
Thurs:	Fri:
Pre-Race Nutrition:	
Goals for the Next Race:	

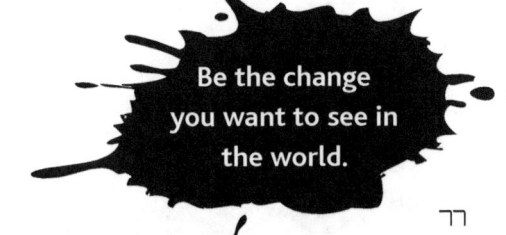

Be the change you want to see in the world.

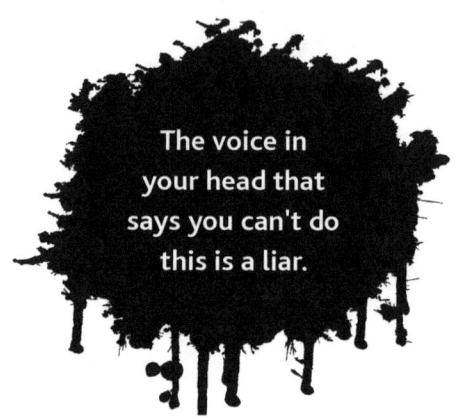

The voice in your head that says you can't do this is a liar.

 Racing Tip:
Run your own race, not that of the person next to you.

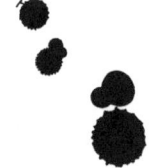

MUD & OBSTACLE RACE LOGBOOK

Race Name:	
Bib #:	Date:
Rating: ☆☆☆☆☆	Difficulty: 💀💀💀💀💀
Location:	Wave Start Time:
Race Length:	Num Obstacles:
My Run Time:	Partner/Team:
Favorite Obstacles:	

Strengths & Weaknesses:

New Friends: (Name, Email, Facebook, Twitter)

Race Comments: (Course, Performance, Party, Injury)

Pre-Race Training

Sun:	Mon:
Tues:	Wed:
Thurs:	Fri:

Pre-Race Nutrition:

Goals for the Next Race:

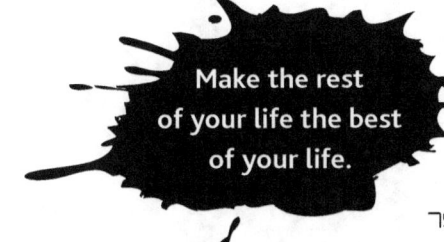

Make the rest of your life the best of your life.

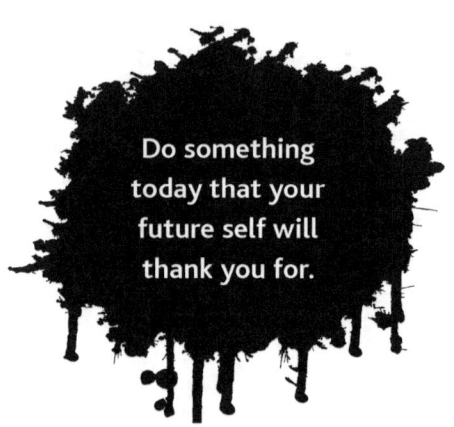

Do something today that your future self will thank you for.

 Racing Tip:
We have all forgotten to fuel, hydrate, stretch, and apply sunblock before a race. But we run anyway.

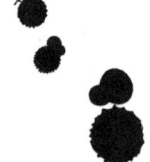

MUD & OBSTACLE RACE LOGBOOK

Race Name:	
Bib #:	Date:
Rating: ☆☆☆☆☆	Difficulty: 💀💀💀💀💀
Location:	Wave Start Time:
Race Length:	Num Obstacles:
My Run Time:	Partner/Team:
Favorite Obstacles:	

Strengths & Weaknesses:

New Friends: (Name, Email, Facebook, Twitter)

Race Comments: (Course, Performance, Party, Injury)

Pre-Race Training

Sun:	Mon:
Tues:	Wed:
Thurs:	Fri:
Pre-Race Nutrition:	

Goals for the Next Race:

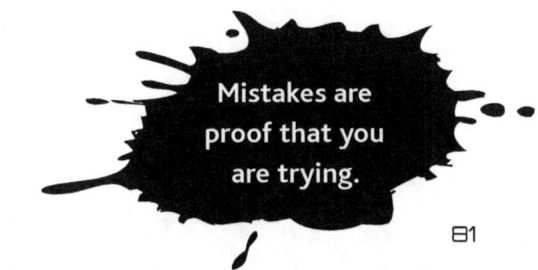

Mistakes are proof that you are trying.

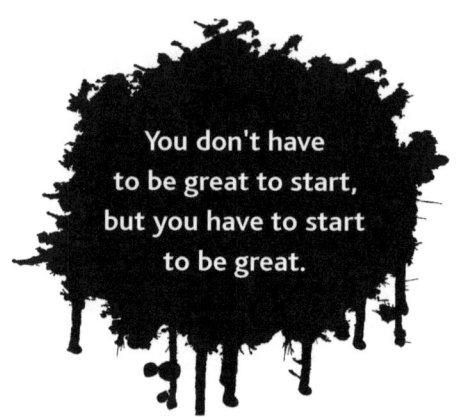

You don't have to be great to start, but you have to start to be great.

 Racing Tip:
If the race is longer than one hour carry some fuel in the form of fruit sauce, gel, or gu packets.

Race Name:	
Bib #:	Date:
Rating: ☆☆☆☆☆	Difficulty: 💀💀💀💀💀
Location:	Wave Start Time:
Race Length:	Num Obstacles:
My Run Time:	Partner/Team:
Favorite Obstacles:	
Strengths & Weaknesses:	
New Friends: (Name, Email, Facebook, Twitter)	
Race Comments: (Course, Performance, Party, Injury)	

Pre-Race Training

Sun:	Mon:
Tues:	Wed:
Thurs:	Fri:
Pre-Race Nutrition:	
Goals for the Next Race:	

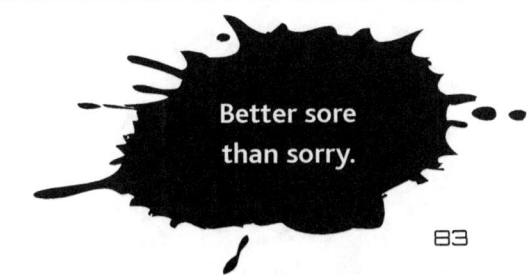

Better sore than sorry.

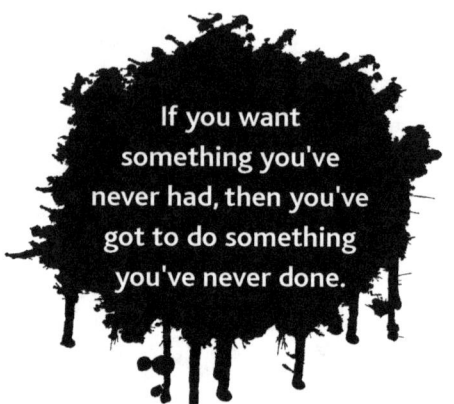

If you want something you've never had, then you've got to do something you've never done.

 Racing Tip:

For rope climbing and hoisting buckets of gravel, look for the thickest rope. Thin ropes take more strength to grip than fat ropes.

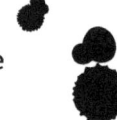

Race Name:	
Bib #:	Date:
Rating: ☆☆☆☆☆	Difficulty: ☠☠☠☠☠
Location:	Wave Start Time:
Race Length:	Num Obstacles:
My Run Time:	Partner/Team:
Favorite Obstacles:	
Strengths & Weaknesses:	
New Friends: (Name, Email, Facebook, Twitter)	
Race Comments: (Course, Performance, Party, Injury)	

Pre-Race Training

Sun:	Mon:
Tues:	Wed:
Thurs:	Fri:
Pre-Race Nutrition:	
Goals for the Next Race:	

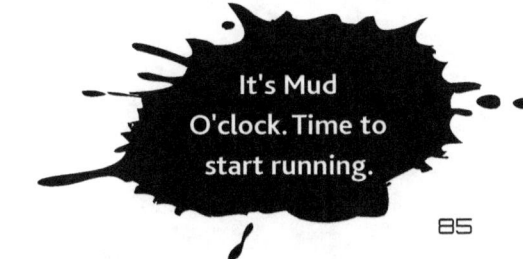

It's Mud O'clock. Time to start running.

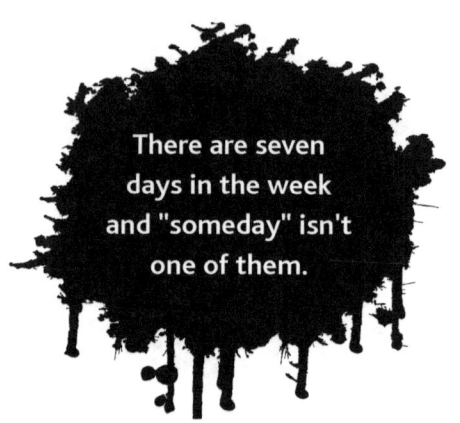

There are seven days in the week and "someday" isn't one of them.

 Racing Tip:
Before throwing the spear, balance the middle of the spear in your hand, then move your hand back about 6 inches. This will keep the point down and level.

MUD & OBSTACLE RACE LOGBOOK

Race Name:	
Bib #:	Date:
Rating: ☆☆☆☆☆	Difficulty: 💀💀💀💀💀
Location:	Wave Start Time:
Race Length:	Num Obstacles:
My Run Time:	Partner/Team:
Favorite Obstacles:	
Strengths & Weaknesses:	
New Friends: (Name, Email, Facebook, Twitter)	
Race Comments: (Course, Performance, Party, Injury)	

Pre-Race Training

Sun:	Mon:
Tues:	Wed:
Thurs:	Fri:
Pre-Race Nutrition:	
Goals for the Next Race:	

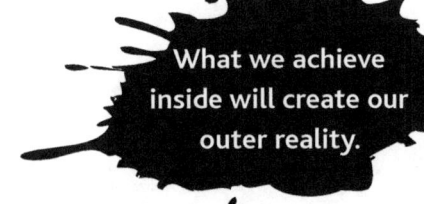

What we achieve inside will create our outer reality.

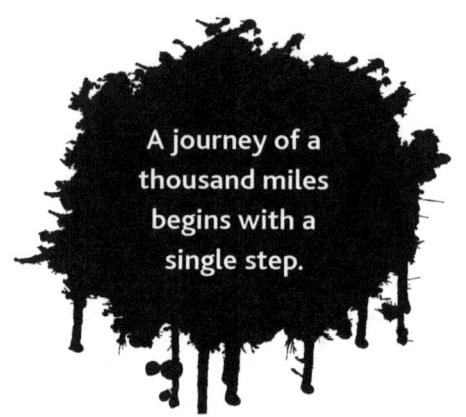

A journey of a thousand miles begins with a single step.

 Racing Tip:
If you have to do burpees for failing an obstacle, loop back afterward and practice the obstacle again. This is the best time to learn.

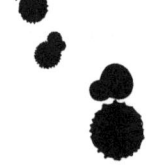

MUD & OBSTACLE RACE LOGBOOK

Race Name:	
Bib #:	Date:
Rating: ☆☆☆☆☆	Difficulty: 💀💀💀💀💀
Location:	Wave Start Time:
Race Length:	Num Obstacles:
My Run Time:	Partner/Team:
Favorite Obstacles:	
Strengths & Weaknesses:	
New Friends: (Name, Email, Facebook, Twitter)	
Race Comments: (Course, Performance, Party, Injury)	

Pre-Race Training

Sun:	Mon:
Tues:	Wed:
Thurs:	Fri:
Pre-Race Nutrition:	
Goals for the Next Race:	

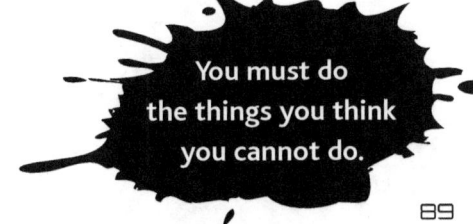

You must do the things you think you cannot do.

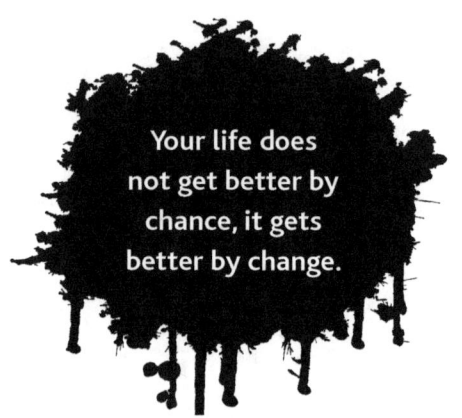

Your life does not get better by chance, it gets better by change.

 Racing Tip:
Once you have mastered the rope climb, try flipping over and ringing the bell with your foot. It is a real crowd pleaser.

Race Name:	
Bib #:	Date:
Rating: ☆☆☆☆☆	Difficulty: 💀💀💀💀💀
Location:	Wave Start Time:
Race Length:	Num Obstacles:
My Run Time:	Partner/Team:
Favorite Obstacles:	

Strengths & Weaknesses:

New Friends: (Name, Email, Facebook, Twitter)

Race Comments: (Course, Performance, Party, Injury)

Pre-Race Training

Sun:	Mon:
Tues:	Wed:
Thurs:	Fri:
Pre-Race Nutrition:	
Goals for the Next Race:	

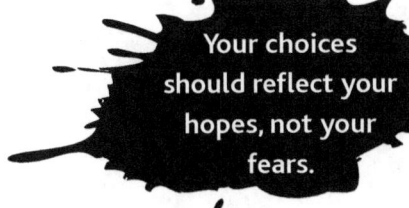

Your choices should reflect your hopes, not your fears.

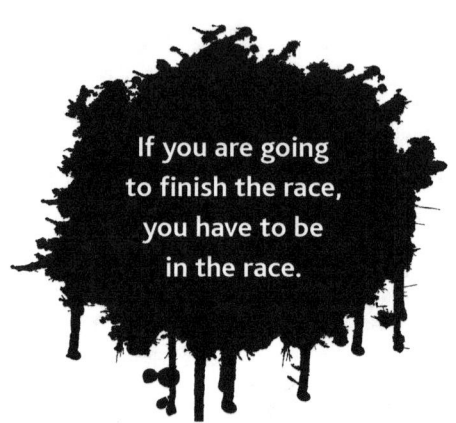

If you are going to finish the race, you have to be in the race.

 Racing Tip:
Crawling under barbed wire is a lot easier if you tuck your arms to your chest and roll sideways. It is faster and consumes less than half as much energy.

MUD & OBSTACLE RACE LOGBOOK

Race Name:	
Bib #:	Date:
Rating: ☆☆☆☆☆	Difficulty: 💀💀💀💀💀
Location:	Wave Start Time:
Race Length:	Num Obstacles:
My Run Time:	Partner/Team:
Favorite Obstacles:	
Strengths & Weaknesses:	
New Friends: (Name, Email, Facebook, Twitter)	
Race Comments: (Course, Performance, Party, Injury)	

Pre-Race Training

Sun:	Mon:
Tues:	Wed:
Thurs:	Fri:
Pre-Race Nutrition:	
Goals for the Next Race:	

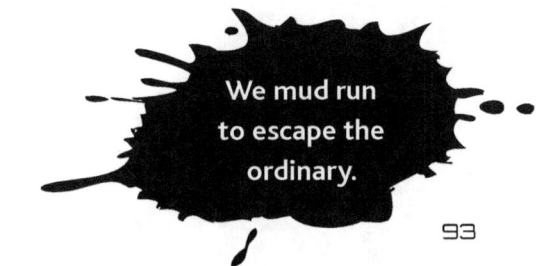

We mud run to escape the ordinary.

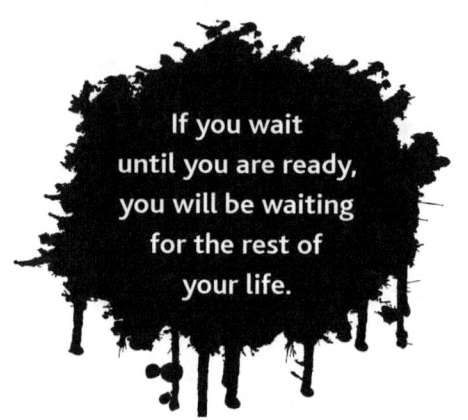

If you wait
until you are ready,
you will be waiting
for the rest of
your life.

 Racing Tip:
Anytime you come to a water station, take water. Don't wait until you feel thirsty before you start drinking.

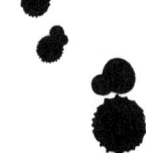

Race Name:	
Bib #:	Date:
Rating: ☆☆☆☆☆	Difficulty: 💀💀💀💀💀
Location:	Wave Start Time:
Race Length:	Num Obstacles:
My Run Time:	Partner/Team:

Favorite Obstacles:

Strengths & Weaknesses:

New Friends: (Name, Email, Facebook, Twitter)

Race Comments: (Course, Performance, Party, Injury)

Pre-Race Training

Sun:	Mon:
Tues:	Wed:
Thurs:	Fri:

Pre-Race Nutrition:

Goals for the Next Race:

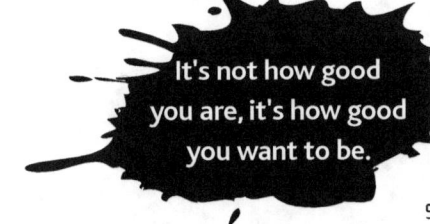

It's not how good you are, it's how good you want to be.

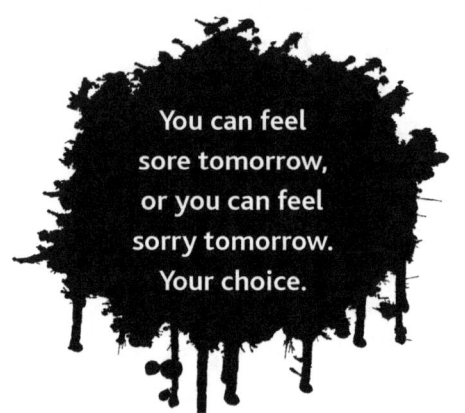

You can feel sore tomorrow, or you can feel sorry tomorrow. Your choice.

 Racing Tip:
If deep mud threatens to take your shoes, point your toes down and walk like a ballerina.

Race Name:	
Bib #:	Date:
Rating: ☆☆☆☆☆	Difficulty: ☠☠☠☠☠
Location:	Wave Start Time:
Race Length:	Num Obstacles:
My Run Time:	Partner/Team:
Favorite Obstacles:	
Strengths & Weaknesses:	
New Friends: (Name, Email, Facebook, Twitter)	
Race Comments: (Course, Performance, Party, Injury)	

Pre-Race Training

Sun:	Mon:
Tues:	Wed:
Thurs:	Fri:
Pre-Race Nutrition:	
Goals for the Next Race:	

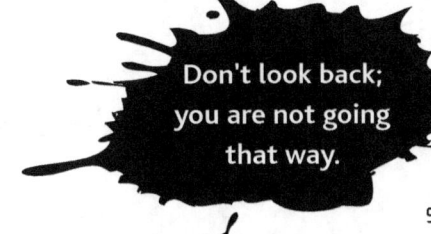

Don't look back; you are not going that way.

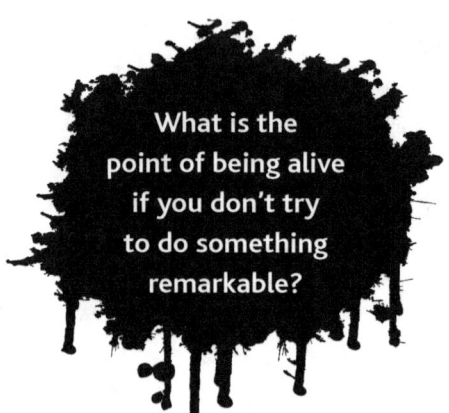

What is the
point of being alive
if you don't try
to do something
remarkable?

 Racing Tip:
When jumping from a tower
into water, shouting "Geronimo"
always makes it easier. That is why
paratroopers do it.

Race Name:	
Bib #:	Date:
Rating: ☆☆☆☆☆	Difficulty: 💀💀💀💀💀
Location:	Wave Start Time:
Race Length:	Num Obstacles:
My Run Time:	Partner/Team:

Favorite Obstacles:

Strengths & Weaknesses:

New Friends: (Name, Email, Facebook, Twitter)

Race Comments: (Course, Performance, Party, Injury)

Pre-Race Training

Sun:	Mon:
Tues:	Wed:
Thurs:	Fri:

Pre-Race Nutrition:

Goals for the Next Race:

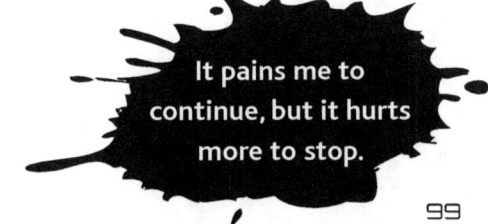

It pains me to continue, but it hurts more to stop.

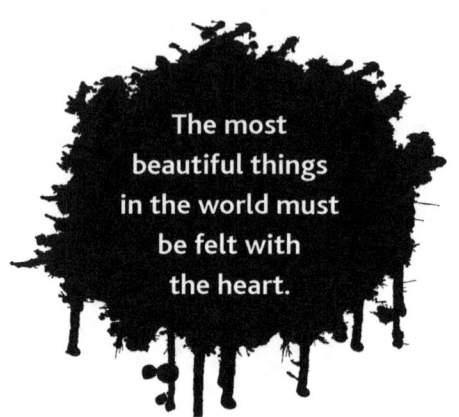

The most beautiful things in the world must be felt with the heart.

 Racing Tip:
Do not grip a monkey bar like a baseball bat. Make your fingers and thumb into a single hook that curls over the bar.

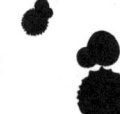

MUD & OBSTACLE RACE LOGBOOK

Race Name:	
Bib #:	Date:
Rating: ☆☆☆☆☆	Difficulty: 💀💀💀💀💀
Location:	Wave Start Time:
Race Length:	Num Obstacles:
My Run Time:	Partner/Team:
Favorite Obstacles:	

Strengths & Weaknesses:

New Friends: (Name, Email, Facebook, Twitter)

Race Comments: (Course, Performance, Party, Injury)

Pre-Race Training

Sun:	Mon:
Tues:	Wed:
Thurs:	Fri:
Pre-Race Nutrition:	

Goals for the Next Race:

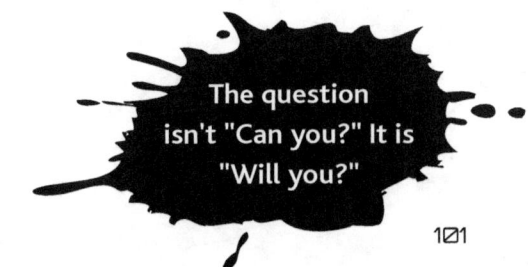

The question isn't "Can you?" It is "Will you?"

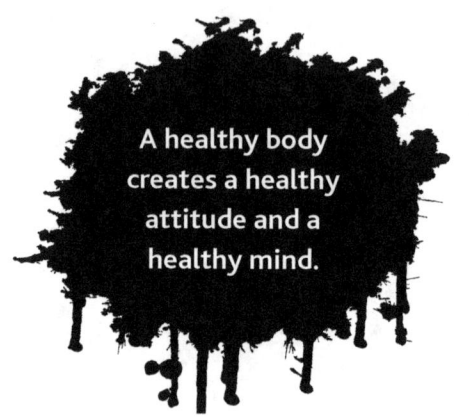

A healthy body creates a healthy attitude and a healthy mind.

 Racing Tip:
When a water obstacle reaches knee deep, slow to a walk. The energy required to run is too great and will wear you down.

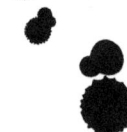

MUD & OBSTACLE RACE LOGBOOK

Race Name:	
Bib #:	Date:
Rating: ☆☆☆☆☆	Difficulty: 💀💀💀💀💀
Location:	Wave Start Time:
Race Length:	Num Obstacles:
My Run Time:	Partner/Team:

Favorite Obstacles:

Strengths & Weaknesses:

New Friends: (Name, Email, Facebook, Twitter)

Race Comments: (Course, Performance, Party, Injury)

Pre-Race Training

Sun:	Mon:
Tues:	Wed:
Thurs:	Fri:

Pre-Race Nutrition:

Goals for the Next Race:

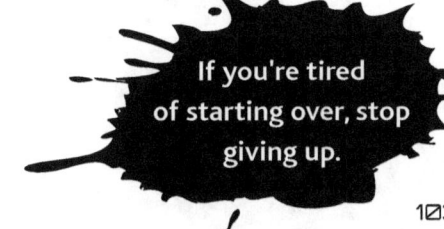

If you're tired of starting over, stop giving up.

www.ingramcontent.com/pod-product-compliance
Lightning Source LLC
Chambersburg PA
CBHW052213090526
44584CB00017BB/2297